healing
massage

**Denise Whichello Brown B.Sc.,
Cert. Ed., D.O., M.I.F.P.A., M.I.F.R.**

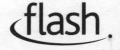

For UK order enquiries: please contact Bookpoint Ltd, 130 Milton Park, Abingdon, Oxon OX14 4SB. *Telephone*: +44 (0) 1235 827720. *Fax*: +44 (0) 1235 400454. Lines are open 09.00–17.00, Monday to Saturday, with a 24-hour message answering service. Details about our titles and how to order are available at www.hoddereducation.com

British Library Cataloguing in Publication Data: a catalogue record for this title is available from the British Library.

First published in UK 2011 by Hodder Education, part of Hachette UK, 338 Euston Road, London NW1 3BH.

Copyright © 2011 Denise Whichello Brown

In UK: All rights reserved. Apart from any permitted use under UK copyright law, no part of this publication may be reproduced or transmitted in any form or by any means, electronic or mechanical, including photocopy, recording, or any information, storage and retrieval system, without permission in writing from the publisher or under licence from the Copyright Licensing Agency Limited. Further details of such licences (for reprographic reproduction) may be obtained from the Copyright Licensing Agency Limited, of Saffron House, 6–10 Kirby Street, London EC1N 8TS.

Typeset by MPS Limited, a Macmillan Company.

Printed in Great Britain for Hodder Education, an Hachette UK Company, 338 Euston Road, London NW1 3BH, by CPI Cox & Wyman, Reading, Berkshire RG1 8EX.

The publisher has used its best endeavours to ensure that the URLs for external websites referred to in this book are correct and active at the time of going to press. However, the publisher and the author have no responsibility for the websites and can make no guarantee that a site will remain live or that the content will remain relevant, decent or appropriate.

Hachette UK's policy is to use papers that are natural, renewable and recyclable products and made from wood grown in sustainable forests. The logging and manufacturing processes are expected to conform to the environmental regulations of the country of origin.

Impression number   10 9 8 7 6 5 4 3 2 1

Year   2015 2014 2013 2012 2011

Contents

Introduction

Massage is an instinctive therapy that everyone has the ability to learn. The aim of this book is to encourage your natural abilities to practise safely and effectively on your family and friends.

You employ your innate ability to touch therapeutically in your daily life. If you have a headache, you instinctively rub around the neck and the temples to soothe away the pain and tension. If you hurt your knee or bang your elbow, your first reaction is to massage it to relieve the pain. Children will hold and rub their tummies when they have stomach ache and eventually the pain will go. A parent feels a child's feverish forehead to check for a high temperature and will massage in response to a child's bumps and cries of pain.

The healing power of therapeutic massage is also used for emotional problems. To comfort distraught friends or relatives you may put your arms around them, hold or stroke them to comfort, support and reassure them in their times of need.

Body and mind should not be regarded as separate entities. Physical symptoms such as headaches or constant fatigue are often an indication of what is 'on our mind'. Muscles contract and tighten in response to anger and anxiety or may become slack as we resign ourselves to what is happening in our lives. Within the physical body is buried a whole lifetime of experience and emotions – birth, childhood, pleasure and pain, shock, frustration, fear, grief, joy and much more besides. Massage is an excellent tool for enabling us to become more aware of what is happening deep within us.

The importance and need for touch is reflected in our everyday language. We talk of being 'deeply touched' when trying to express a reaction. We ask our friends to 'keep in touch' or 'stay in contact' with us. We speak of 'being in touch' or 'out of touch' with our feelings. We describe others as being a 'soft touch' or a bit 'touchy'. We also experience 'gut feelings' about a particular situation.

Touch is essential for our growth and well-being. It is the first sense to be developed in the womb, and early touching while the foetus grows in the womb enhances the development of the nervous system and encourages communication and close bonding between mother and baby. Children need cuddles from their parents to give them a feeling of security and to show them how much they are loved.

setting the
scene

It is important to create the perfect ambience for your healing massage. Although you may have to improvise in places that are not ideal it is important to pay attention to the surroundings and make sure you have everything you need close at hand. If you set the scene carefully your friends and family will derive maximum benefit from your treatments.

It is very beneficial to use carrier oils for your healing massage. It's important to choose cold-pressed, unrefined and additive-free oils full of vitamins and minerals to nourish and revitalize the skin.

Although massage is very safe there are some occasions when care needs to be taken, and this chapter will make you aware of these.

Environment

Careful preparation and the right setting will make a good massage even better! Both the giver and receiver should feel relaxed as soon as they arrive. Always ensure that all towels, cushions and oils are on hand so that you will not lose contact and thus break the flow of the massage. A massage should never be hurried.

To carry out a massage you will need:
* a thick duvet or a large piece of foam for your massage partner to lie on (or massage couch)
* three large towels
* three pillows/cushions
* carrier oil (e.g. sweet almond).

Peace and quiet

These are vital. Ensure that you choose a time when you will not be disturbed. Intrusions and distractions are extremely disconcerting, breaking your concentration and destroying the flow of your massage movements. Take the telephone off the hook and tell your friends and family not to enter the room. You may decide to choose some soothing background music, although this is a matter of personal preference. Some people will prefer silence.

Cleanliness

Always wash your hands before as well as after the treatment. Make sure that your fingernails are short and clean – trim them as far down as possible. Do not wear any jewellery on your hands. Rings, bracelets and watches can all scratch the receiver.

Warmth

The room should be draught-free and warm, yet well ventilated. Nothing will destroy a massage more quickly than physical coldness; it is impossible to relax when you feel cold. Heat the room prior to treatment and, as the receiver's body temperature will drop, ensure that you have a good supply of towels. Keep all parts of the receiver's body covered other than the area on which you are working. Warm your hands if they feel cold, either by rubbing them briskly together, or by immersing them in warm water.

Lighting

Soft and subdued lighting will create the ideal atmosphere. Bright lights falling on the receiver's face will not make for a relaxing atmosphere and will cause tension around the eyes. Candlelight provides the perfect setting, or you may wish to use a tinted bulb. Choose colours such as pale pink, blue, green, peach or lavender.

Colour

The most therapeutic colours to have in the room are pastel shades – pale pink, blue, green, lilac or peach decor and towels are perfect for the occasion. Colours such as red will tend to generate anger and restlessness.

Clothes

Wear comfortable and loose-fitting clothes as you need to move around easily and the room in which you will be working will be warm. White is the best colour to wear when giving a massage since it will deflect away any negativity (negative emotions) released from the individual being treated. Go barefoot if possible, otherwise wear flat shoes. The receiver should undress down to whatever level is comfortable. Suggest he or she undresses down to at least underwear. Point out that any areas which are not being worked on will be covered up as this will create a sense of security and trust.

To prepare yourself to give a massage:
* wear comfortable and loose-fitting clothes
* make sure your fingernails are short and clean
* remove all jewellery
* wash your hands.

Finishing touches

Fresh flowers will scent your room or you could burn some incense or essential oils before the treatment. Refer to Chapter 4, where 16 essential oils are explained, for suggestions. Crystals may also enhance the environment. Rose quartz relaxes and soothes and amethyst is useful for absorbing both physical and emotional negativity. At the end of the treatment a piece of obsidian, haematite, black tourmaline or smoky quartz can be used to 'ground' the receiver.

Equipment

Massage surface

You may work on the floor using a firm yet well-padded surface. This will allow you to give a massage wherever you want. Place a large, thick piece of foam, or two or three blankets, or a thick duvet on the floor. Use plenty of cushions during the massage.

When the receiver is lying on the back (supine position), place one cushion under the head and one under the knees to take the pressure off the lower back.

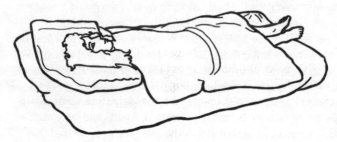

Figure 1.1 *Working with receiver lying on the back.*

When the receiver is lying on the front (prone position), place a cushion under the feet, one under the head and shoulders and one under the abdomen if you wish.

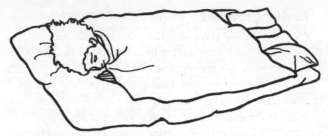

Figure 1.2 *Working with receiver lying on the front.*

Ensure that you have something to kneel on to avoid sore knees. If you are unfortunate enough to suffer from a bad back or have knee problems, it may be a good idea to invest in a portable couch. It is far less tiring and you can reach the receiver's body more easily. You could improvise by using the kitchen table, if the height is comfortable for you.

Never use a bed to give a massage as most are far too soft and wide for massage purposes and any pressure you apply will be absorbed by the mattress. Also, a bed will not be the right height for your back.

Carrier oils

I believe that the only really effective way to massage is with oil. Your hands will glide smoothly over the skin and the movements will flow freely. In addition, oil massage makes the skin smooth and soft.

The carrier oil (also known as base oil or fixed oil) you choose should always be of vegetable origin and also cold pressed (not removed by chemicals), unrefined and additive free. Cold pressed, unrefined carrier oils contain vitamins, minerals and fatty acids and, therefore, nourish the skin. The more highly processed the vegetable oils are, the less vitamin content will be retained. I do not recommend the use of mineral oil, such as commercial baby oil, because it is not easily absorbed. Vegetable oil molecules are easily absorbed through the skin pores, whereas mineral oil tends to clog the pores.

It is a good idea to mix several different base oils together for a therapeutic formula. The lighter vegetable oils may be used unblended if you wish (e.g. sweet almond, apricot kernel, peach kernel, grapeseed) or they may constitute the highest proportion of the massage blend. The thicker, richer oils, which are usually more expensive, may be added to improve absorption and nourish the skin. The thicker oils tend to be too heavy and sticky when used on their own in a full treatment.

This is my favourite recipe for a special carrier oil blend:

The carrier oils in my 'special blend' are all highly therapeutic in their own right.

To a 100 ml bottle add:
* one teaspoon (approximately 5 ml) apricot kernel oil
* one teaspoon avocado pear oil
* one teaspoon calendula oil
* one teaspoon evening primrose oil
* one teaspoon jojoba oil
* one teaspoon peach kernel oil
* one teaspoon wheatgerm oil
* fill up the bottle with sweet almond oil.

Sweet almond oil (*Prunus amygdalis*)

Contains many vitamins, minerals and fatty acids and is useful for all skin types. It is particularly good for dry, sensitive, inflamed or prematurely aged skin. It can be used on its own as a base oil. Sweet almond oil is popular and is often used as the highest proportion of a massage blend. It is a pale yellow, low-odour oil much favoured by the beauty industry – it was used by Napoleon's wife Josephine!

Apricot kernel (*Prunus armenica*) and peach kernel oil (*Prunus persica*)

Excellent for all skin types. Their nourishing properties make them an ideal choice for a facial oil, particularly where the skin is dry or sensitive. Although I add them to my blend they could be used unblended, although they are more expensive than sweet almond oil as they are produced in smaller quantities.

Avocado pear oil (*Persea americana*)

Has a wonderful dark green colour if it is unrefined and contains vitamin D, lecithin and fatty acids. It penetrates well in spite of its thickness, and is healing and soothing for all skin types. Dry, dehydrated skin, wrinkled skin and eczema particularly will benefit. It normally constitutes ten per cent or less of a blend.

Calendula oil (*Calendula officinalis*)

Has anti-inflammatory, astringent, hormonal, healing and soothing properties. It is particularly suitable for eczema, psoriasis, rashes, broken and thread veins, varicose veins, wounds, scars, bedsores, bruises and sensitive skin. Calendula cream is popular among homoeopaths. Calendula oil would normally make up ten per cent of a blend.

Evening primrose oil (*Oenothera biennis*)

Increasingly popular, although it is expensive. It contains a therapeutic ingredient known as gamma linoleic acid (GLA) as well as vitamins and minerals. It is recommended for relieving PMS (pre-menstrual syndrome), menopausal problems, MS (multiple sclerosis), heart disease, high cholesterol levels, eczema and psoriasis. It is excellent for regenerating and stimulating the skin. Normally up to ten per cent is used in a blend. Evening primrose oil is often administered internally in capsule form.

Jojoba oil (*Simmondsia chinensis*)

A thick, yellow oil rich in protein and minerals. It nourishes, moisturizes and penetrates deeply and is wonderful as a face or a hair oil. Acne, eczema, dry skin conditions, inflammatory conditions, psoriasis and indeed all skin types will derive benefit from jojoba oil. As a rule up to a ten per cent blend is used.

Wheatgerm oil (*Triticum vulgare*)

A rich, orange-brown colour oil, invaluable to any blend. It is anti-oxidant and, therefore, prevents the oil from becoming rancid. An ideal preservative. It contains protein, minerals, vitamins and is particularly renowned for its vitamin E content. Its nourishing properties are useful to combat prematurely ageing skin, eczema and psoriasis. It also helps to prevent stretch marks. It is usually added up to ten per cent in a blend.

Buying base oils

Carrier oils vary widely in price: evening primrose oil costs far more than sweet almond oil.

Always look for 'cold pressed' vegetable carrier oils. The virgin oil is of the highest quality as it comes from the first pressing and has the highest vitamin and mineral content. After the first pressing, the base oil may be treated with heat or synthetically to remove colour or aroma and the vitamin and mineral content will be drastically reduced. The best base oils which are 'cold pressed' will usually have a rich colour and a characteristic aroma.

Pure essential oils may be added to the carrier oil in order to enhance the treatment (see Chapter 5 and also my other book, *Flash: Natural Healing with Aromatherapy*).

When blending essential oils with a carrier oil, the essential oil content is usually between one per cent and three per cent. Approximately 20 drops of essential oil is equivalent to 1 ml. Therefore, a 1.5 per cent essential oil content which I recommend would be:

* 3 drops to 10 mls
* 15 drops to 50 mls
* 30 drops to 100 mls

How to use base oils

Always keep the oil within easy reach during the treatment. Do not use too much oil as you will be unable to make proper contact and the receiver will feel most uncomfortable and sticky. A complete treatment actually requires only a few teaspoons of oil. Warm the oil before the massage.

Never pour oil directly onto the body. Pour about 2 ml (half a teaspoon) onto the palm of one hand and then rub your hands together to warm the oil slightly before applying it. When you require more lubricant keep one hand in contact with the body. Breaking contact destroys the continuity of the massage and creates a feeling of insecurity.

Contraindications (when not to massage)

Some contraindications are **total** when massage should never be performed. Other contraindications are **local** when massage can be performed over the rest of the body but not over the contraindicated areas.

Massage is generally very safe but if there is a serious medical condition present, or if you are in any doubt then do ask a medically qualified doctor. **If in doubt – check it out!**

High temperature/fevers

The body is already fighting off toxins as indicated by the rise in temperature. A massage would release even more unwelcome toxins into the system. This is a total contraindication.

Infectious and contagious diseases

These include ringworm, scabies, impetigo and chicken pox – you do not want to spread the condition or transfer it to yourself. This is a total contraindication.

Under the influence of drugs or after heavy drinking

This is a total contraindication.

Thrombophlebitis and other similar conditions

Phlebitis is inflammation of a vein. The skin near the inflamed vein is red, hot and swollen. If a clot (thrombus) forms in the vein, massage is contraindicated since the clot could move. This is a total contraindication.

Advanced varicose veins

You risk the danger here of causing further inflammation and great pain. Totally avoid advanced varicose veins, be cautious with minor varicose veins.

Recent scars or operations

Beware of recent scars and open wounds. This is a local contraindication. Old scar tissue can be massaged.

Abdomen during pregnancy

Although massage is extremely beneficial during pregnancy, only light massage should be applied to the abdominal area. All other areas can be massaged in the normal way. Where there is a history of risk of miscarriage take particular care during the first three months.

Undiagnosed lumps, bumps and moles

These may be innocent but it is wise to have them investigated by a medically qualified doctor. This is a local contraindication.

Cuts, wounds, bites, bruises or sunburn

Any of these areas should be avoided. This is a local contraindication.

Inflammatory conditions e.g. bursitis (housemaid's knee)

Signs of inflammation include redness, heat, swelling, tenderness, pain and loss of movement. Inflamed organs should also never be massaged (e.g. gastroenteritis). This is a local contraindication.

Cancer and massage

There is a great deal of confusion and fear surrounding massage and cancer, and there are still many questions that need to be answered. It is interesting that some oncology (cancer) units in hospitals now have massage therapists. It is no longer the case that massage is only offered in hospices at the final stages of cancer. In cancer patients, gentle massage will have many benefits. Aches and pains may be considerably relieved as the body produces endorphins (pain relievers) in response to the stimulus of touch. Stress, tension and insomnia may be relieved and after a good night's sleep it is much easier to cope and put things in perspective. Anticipatory nausea evoked by the fear and dread prior to chemotherapy can be helped by massage given before the treatment.

Massage encourages a positive body image – a woman who has had a mastectomy may feel unfeminine and disfigured; massage will allow her to feel a whole person once again.

Constipation, a common side effect of the opiate group of painkillers, such as codeine, can also be alleviated by the use of abdominal massage (**unless there is active disease in this area**).

massage techniques

The classical massage movements are effleurage, friction, petrissage, percussion and vibration. Each one has clear therapeutic effects; of course, there are also common errors that should be avoided.

Even though there are a wide variety of different massage movements, most techniques are merely a variation on the strokes described in the section. With the aid of these fundamental movements you will be able to perform a complete body massage.

Don't try and do too much or learn too much at once. It's not necessary to master all the massage movements in a single session. Start by practising just one or two movements and you will be amazed at how quickly your massage movements begin to flow. As you develop and gain confidence, you will begin to invent your own strokes and build up an extensive repertoire. Be guided by your hands; be spontaneous and develop your own individual massage style.

Effleurage/Stroking

The word effleurage is derived from the French 'effleurer' – to stroke/touch lightly. It is one of the principal movements of massage and may be performed on any area of the body. It signals the beginning and the end of a massage both preceding and succeeding all other strokes and facilitating the flow from one movement to the next.

Description

To practise effleurage on the back make sure your massage partner is comfortable and then draw the top towel down to expose the back and tuck it into the underwear.

Position yourself comfortably at the side of the receiver. Put a small amount of oil onto one hand, rub your hands briskly together to warm the oil and then place both hands, flat down, at the bottom of the back, one either side of the spine.

Stroke up the entire length of the back and across the shoulders and then glide gently back down to your starting point with a feather-light touch. Repeat these stroking movements until your movements feel smooth and flowing.

Use the palms and fingers of both hands as you glide over the surface of the skin moulding your hands to the contours of the body. You should keep as much of the hands as possible in contact with the body. The receiver experiences one continuous movement as you apply firm rhythmic pressure on the upward stroke yet glide lightly downwards to your starting point (see Figure 2.1). Maintain an even rhythm and avoid jerky movements at all times. Pressure can be superficial or deep according to the effect required. Close your eyes as you effleurage to accentuate and heighten your sensitivity and sense of touch. Experiment with different depths of pressure. To achieve a firmer pressure use your body weight to lean into the movement. As you practise on different people you will find some people prefer firm effleurage whereas others will like gentle stroking.

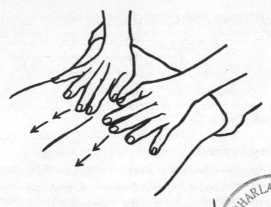

Figure 2.1 *Effleurage of the back.*

Therapeutic effects

* Effleurage enables you to distribute the massage oil.
* The receiver experiences an immediate sense of well-being and relaxation.
* A relationship of trust is established between the two of you as your hands become accustomed to the receiver's body.
* It enables you to familiarize yourself with the amount of pressure to apply.
* It provides a link between techniques.
* It prepares the body for deeper movements.
* Effleurage, when performed slowly, has a sedative action and is particularly beneficial for soothing the nerves. Stress and strain may be relieved, tension headaches dispelled and patterns of insomnia broken.
* Brisk effleurage enlivens, revives and stimulates the central nervous system.
* The tissues will warm up as you stroke the body, improving the circulation.
* The flow of lymph is increased, helping to get rid of waste and poisonous substances.

* Effleurage improves the skin since it helps desquamation (removal of dead skin cells), encouraging a healthy and glowing complexion.
* It enables you to detect any areas that may be tighter than others.

Errors to avoid

* Do not lose contact with the receiver (loss of contact means loss of confidence and loss of relaxation).
* Relax your hands and flow, avoiding any jerky or sudden movements (jerky movements cause jangled nerves). The movements must be rhythmic, smooth and even.
* Use your whole hand and not just the fingertips (you can cover a much wider area), except when working on small areas such as the face.
* Remember, no pressure whatsoever on the downward stroke. Effleurage is always performed towards the heart – up the legs, and arms, and up the back. It can also be applied in a centripetal direction (in a circle travelling towards the centre) or in a centrifugal direction (in a circle travelling outwards away from the centre).

> **Remember!** If in doubt, effleurage! Everyone adores this stroke.

Friction

The word friction is derived from the Latin 'fricare' – to rub. This is a deep technique particularly useful for breaking down knots and nodules in muscles and for loosening tightness around joints.

Description

Friction movements normally make use of the balls of the thumbs (although the fingertips, knuckles or even the elbows may be used). The muscle is moved against the bone by small circular movements of the balls of the thumbs. You stand directly over the area to be treated and use your body weight to penetrate right down into the deeper tissues – the human body is not as delicate and fragile as you might imagine.

This stroke is particularly effective when performed on either side of the spine (see Figure 2.2). If your thumbs are not aching by the time you reach the neck area you are not performing the stroke correctly! However, your thumbs will quickly become used to friction.

To practise friction on the back, position yourself at the side of the receiver and do not use too much oil otherwise your thumbs will slide around and you will find it more difficult to locate the knots.

Place the pads of your thumbs in the dimples located either side of the base of the spine. Work from the dimples up towards the base of the neck using small, slow, deep circular outward friction movements. Then glide gently back down to your starting point.

Slowly friction up the back again and this time try to find some knots and nodules. To work on a 'knotty' area place one thumb on top of the other with your fingers splayed out to give support and control. Then move your thumbs slowly over the area in a circular direction. Always friction into an area gradually and ask your

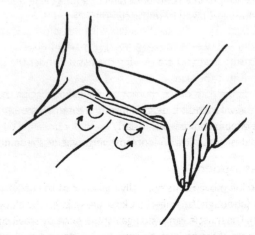

Figure 2.2 *Friction of the back working from the base of the spine towards the neck.*

partner if it feels uncomfortable. A little discomfort is fine but this will feel like a 'good' pain.

Therapeutic effects

* This technique is particularly useful for breaking down the knots and nodules that build up in the body due to the stresses and strains of daily life.
* Any accumulated waste products may be eliminated.
* Friction helps to break down the fatty deposits and is therefore of benefit in cases of obesity.
* Friction is very effective around a **well-healed** scar to break down adhesions.
* It also increases the temperature by increasing cellular activity and bringing an increased flow of blood to an area providing temporary analgesia (pain relief).
* Friction also helps to loosen joints.

Errors to avoid

* Work deeper and deeper into the tissues **gradually**, as the pain tolerance levels vary greatly. Do not over-treat an area as this can lead to pain and soreness.
* Do not hunch your shoulders with the effort (otherwise you will need a massage yourself straight afterwards).
* Ensure that you are moving the tissues under the skin and not just the skin.
* Use the pads of the thumbs only, avoiding digging the nails in!
* Make sure that you are applying the same amount of pressure with both thumbs.
* Never press directly onto the vertebrae of the spine.

Petrissage

Petrissage is derived from the French 'pétrir' meaning to knead. Petrissage can be subdivided into picking-up, squeezing, rolling and wringing. If you are good at kneading dough then you will quickly become an expert!

Description

It is an extremely powerful and vigorous movement, which enables you to work deeply on the muscles. You may apply it to every area of the body, except for the face, and it is effective on the fleshy areas such as the hips and thighs. In **picking-up**, place your hands flat on the part being treated and slowly and carefully grasp the muscle (not the skin) firmly with one or both hands, then lift and stretch the muscle as far away as possible from the bone.

Once you have picked up the muscle you may squeeze it gently. Squeezing is particularly effective in alleviating muscle spasm. You may now roll the muscle in both directions – your thumbs may roll the muscle towards your fingers or your fingers may roll the muscle towards your thumbs. **Wringing** is a variation on picking-up. It is picking-up with a twist! Use alternate hands to pick up the muscle and wring it out. The muscle is picked up and then pulled towards you and 'wrung' out. Imagine that you are wringing out a towel or a chamois leather (see Figure 2.3, showing the technique on a thigh).

To practise petrissage on the leg, position your partner on his/her front.

Cover the back with one towel and use another towel to cover one leg so that only the leg you are working on is exposed. Position yourself at the side of the leg you wish to petrissage. Put a small

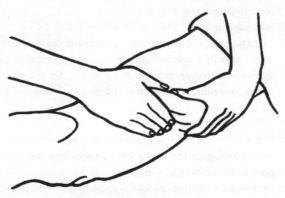

Figure 2.3 *Wringing the back of the thigh.*

amount of oil onto one hand and rub your hands together to warm the oil (take care as too much oil will make it difficult to pick up the muscles).

Place your hands flat down on the calf and gently pick up the muscles away from the bone and squeeze and release several times. Ensure that you are squeezing the muscles and not the skin.

Now try picking up and rolling. Place both hands flat down on the calf and pick up the muscles as before and then roll the muscle taking your thumbs towards the fingers. Repeat several times and then with your hands in the same position as before roll the muscle taking your fingers towards your thumbs.

To perform wringing place both hands flat down on the calf muscles and pick up the muscles with your right hand and grasp and pull towards you, then alternate and use your left hand to grasp and pull the muscles towards you. Try to make your movements rhythmical with no pinching! Now practise your wringing movements on the thigh as in Figure 2.3.

Therapeutic effects

* By alternately squeezing and relaxing, the veins and lymphatic vessels are emptied and filled, bringing fresh nutrients to the muscles.
* Any toxins that have accumulated, such as lactic acid, are removed from the deeper tissues.
* It breaks down tightness in large muscles.
* Petrissage is invaluable in helping to break down and remove fatty deposits around the thighs, shoulders and buttocks.
* It also helps to prevent muscle stiffness after exercise and can relieve muscle spasm and cramp.

Errors to avoid

* Make sure that you use the whole of your hand rather than just your fingers and your thumbs, otherwise there is the danger of pinching the flesh.
* Make sure you are working the muscles and **not** just the skin. Do not just slide over the receiver's skin.

Percussion movements/Tapotement

Percussion is from the Latin 'percutere' which means to hit. It is a stimulating and invigorating technique and involves a series of light, brisk, striking actions applied with alternate hands in rapid succession, performed on large muscle areas to improve circulation and induce muscle tone.

Description

Two of the main percussion strokes are **cupping** and **hacking**; they may be performed on many areas of the body, although they are especially effective when used on fleshy and large muscular areas of the body such as the thighs. Other percussion movements include **flicking, beating** and **pounding** and **tapotement**. When performing percussion movements the action originates from the wrists and not from the elbows or shoulders, which remain still throughout. Many beginners make the mistake of practising percussion movements from the elbows and shoulders, resulting in frustration and clumsiness.

To practise cupping, hacking and flicking on the sides of the back, position yourself at the side of the receiver.

Cupping is performed with your palms facing downwards, forming a hollow curve. It is sometimes known as 'clapping' (see Figure 2.4).

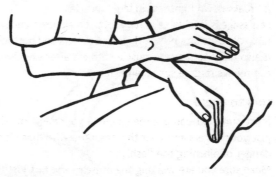

Figure 2.4 *Cupping the sides of the back.*

Form a hollow curve with both hands and hold them, palms down, over the opposite side of the back. Cup up and down the sides of the back paying particular attention to any fleshy areas.

As you bring your cupped hands down on to the body in quick succession, a vacuum is created which is released when you bring your hands up. The sound should be hollow like a horse trotting. Listen for the sound. When you want to cup the other side of the back, position yourself at the other side of your massage partner.

Now try hacking. **Hacking** is probably the best-known massage stroke since it is the movement almost always shown in films. It is achieved with the edge of the hands (the ulnar border). Hold your hands over the opposite side of the lower back with the palms facing each other, the thumbs uppermost (see Figure 2.5). Flick your hands rhythmically up and down in rapid succession, once again working up and down the sides of the back. Use these movements at the end of a massage to wake the person up! Obviously, if you are trying to relax someone hacking may be omitted altogether. If you are nervous about using these movements, practise them first on a cushion or a pillow placed on your lap.

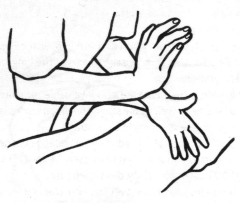

Figure 2.5 *Hacking the sides of the back.*

Let's try flicking too down the sides of the back. **Flicking** is a movement similar to hacking and is often described as 'finger hacking'. To perform this movement flex your wrists slightly and bring ONLY the sides of your little fingers into contact with the body (not the edge of the hands as well). Flicking is a much lighter, softer movement than the usual hacking movement.

Beating and pounding movements are both applied with your hands in a closed position with your fists **lightly** clenched. Beating is performed with the ulnar border (little finger side) of the closed fists, whereas in pounding the palmar surface of the hands are employed. The closed fists are applied to the body in quick succession. Try both these movements over the buttocks to induce muscle tone and break down fatty deposits.

Tapotement is a very gentle form of percussion that uses just the fingertips. It is carried out on delicate areas such as the face. Tapotement is derived from the French 'tapoter' which means to tap or pat. To practise tapotement make sure the fingers are loose and relaxed and gently tap the fingertips all over your face. Why not try tapotement on your partner's face too?

Therapeutic effects

* Percussion movements are very stimulating and extremely useful for athletes before an event.
* As the blood is drawn to the surface the circulation is improved.
* Cupping is beneficial when performed over the upper and middle back area as it loosens mucus in the lungs aiding expectoration.
* Percussion movements are also invaluable for inducing muscle tone as well as for strengthening muscles, since they stimulate the muscle to contract.
* They are also useful for reducing fatty deposits and flabby muscle areas and are often used over the buttocks and thighs. Great for breaking down cellulite!
* Gentle percussion given over the abdomen increases peristalsis, thereby aiding conditions such as constipation.

Errors to avoid

* Make sure that when cupping, your hands are really cupped – otherwise a smacking sound will be heard, which is stinging and painful.
* When hacking do not tense up the fingers of your hands or the movement will feel like a karate chop.
* Keep your hands relaxed and loose and ensure that the movements are coming **from the wrist**. Keep your elbows tucked closely in; if you use your elbows and shoulders you will be exhausted quickly.
* These strokes must not be performed over bony areas such as over the shins – they will hurt.
* Try not to concentrate on the strokes, otherwise you may lose the rhythm.
* Make the movements light and bouncy, not heavy and thumping.

Vibration and shaking

Vibration is a fine, gentle trembling movement of the tissues, which is performed by one or both hand or finger(s). The French word 'vibrer' means to vibrate. **Shaking** is a larger amplitude movement performed more vigorously.

Description

To perform vibration the palmar surface of one or both hands is placed on the part of the body or the limb to be treated and the entire muscle area is vibrated rapidly. The movement may either be gentle, in which case it is known as 'vibration', or vigorous, which is referred to as 'shaking'. Gentle vibration can be performed using just the fingertips along the course of a nerve.

Let's practise vibration on the abdomen. Ask your massage partner to lie on his or her back and remember where to place your pillows – one under the head and one under the knees to take the strain off the lower back. Expose the abdomen only, making sure that all other body parts are covered.

Position yourself to the side of the receiver facing the abdomen. Lower your hands gently down onto the abdomen one on top of the other and then vibrate your hands rapidly yet gently up and down or from side to side. This movement can help to relieve flatulence and constipation.

Therapeutic effects

* Vibration along the course of a nerve is helpful for restoring and maintaining the functions of a nerve and the muscles supplied by them, thereby improving their nutrition. It is particularly useful in cases of paralysis or where there is loss of nerve power.
* Vibration and shaking can be performed on the abdominal area to aid digestion and relieve flatulence. It can be used to promote tone in the colon and to combat constipation and flatulence.
* Vibration and shaking over the thoracic area and chest is particularly beneficial for respiratory problems such as asthma, sometimes in combination with cupping and hacking. It helps to loosen mucus.
* Vibration can also be used to loosen tightness in muscles that are not responding to other movements.

Errors to avoid

* Do not perform vibration and shaking where there is inflammation.
* Do not apply too much pressure.
* Do not lose contact.

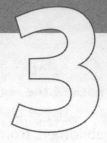

step-by-step massage

A complete full-body massage works on the back of the legs, back, shoulders and neck, face, upper chest and neck, arms and hands, abdomen, front of the legs and feet.

It is easy to carry out a complete treatment on your family and friends. If you do intend to use massage professionally then formal training with a reputable establishment is vital. This will include a thorough grounding in anatomy and physiology, business studies, as well as the completion of case studies.

There is no 'correct' sequence for giving a massage: you may choose to treat the whole body or you may wish to concentrate on just one area – for example, the back.

Ask your massage partner which area(s) they would like you to focus on.

Remember to work intuitively, discovering and experimenting with new techniques to develop your own style.

Before you begin ensure that you have created the right environment and that you have everything you need within easy reach.

Always be aware of your posture. Whether you are working on the floor or at a table, keep your back relaxed yet straight throughout the massage. When standing, bend your knees and tuck your bottom in so that your back can work from a secure base (i.e. the pelvis). Allow your thighs to do most of the work – not your back.

> **Remember!** It should be as relaxing to give a massage as it is to receive one.

With practice you will learn to avoid tensing your muscles so that the healing energy can flow freely through your hands and body. If you do not pay attention to your posture you will quickly become tired. Habits are difficult to break so if you consciously control your posture now instead of slumping it will become automatic later on. Your shoulders, arms and lower back will thus take as little strain as possible. If you are using a couch, stand close to it so that you need only do a minimum amount of reaching.

Ensure that your state of mind is calm when giving a massage. The quality and success of a treatment depends upon this. Do not attempt to give a massage when you are feeling angry, moody, depressed or unwell. Your negativity will be transmitted. Your attention must be devoted entirely to the receiver. If you are worrying about your own problems and your mind is drifting, this will be communicated immediately. Ensure that you are aware of your patient's breathing and that you are sensitive to the receiver's reactions. Observe the facial expressions and be aware of any tensing up in the muscles.

Spend time consciously relaxing yourself before the treatment and, most importantly, be guided by your intuition. Take a few deep breaths before the massage allowing all tension and anxiety to flow out of your body. Breathe in peace and breathe out love. Tune in to the person you are massaging. It may help to work with your eyes closed. Give yourself unselfishly to the massage.

If you are very sensitive and intuitive you may find it helpful to 'ground' yourself prior to a treatment. To 'protect' yourself from any negativity, imagine that white, healing light is pouring down from the sky and protecting you as you work.

You are now ready to begin. Good luck!

Back of the body

Back of the leg (posterior leg massage)

Leg massage is of great benefit, particularly after standing all day at work or after wearing high heels. Leg massage will improve the circulation and help to prevent varicose veins. It is also excellent for the lymphatic system. There may be swelling at the back of the knee (where there are lymph nodes) and also at the ankles. We always massage up the legs towards the lymph glands in the groin area to reduce this fluid. Treatment of the back of the legs often helps to alleviate problems in the lower back. Tightness in the upper thigh muscles is usually linked with low back pain. Leg massage is also useful both as a prelude to exercise and afterwards to prevent stiffness. It's great for cellulite too and for toning muscles.

Remember not to:
* use heavy pressure over varicose veins or where a person has thin skin and/or bruises easily (e.g. diabetics and the elderly)
* use heavy pressure on the delicate area at the back of the knee (the popliteal space)
* work on inflamed or swollen areas
* work over recent scar tissue
* work over infectious skin conditions
* massage where there is thrombophlebitis.

The massage
Position yourself on the side of the leg to be massaged.

1 *Effleuraging the leg*
Put a small amount of oil onto one hand and rub your hands together to warm the oil. Effleurage the entire leg, moulding your hands to the leg. Apply most of the pressure with the palms of your

3 step-by-step massage   **33** hands and hardly any pressure to the back of the knee. Hold your hands in a V-shape with one hand in front of the other or cup your hands to perform the stroking movement (see Figure 3.1). Apply pressure only on the upward movements. Remember that we always massage up the legs, draining towards the lymph glands in the groin. As your hands reach the top of the thigh, separate them and let them glide gently down the sides of the leg to the ankle with no pressure. Gradually increase your upward pressure, but do not press firmly on the delicate area at the back of the knee. Check that your partner is comfortable and ask them if they prefer a firm or a lighter pressure.

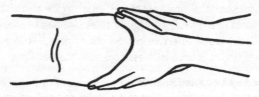

Figure 3.1 *Effleurage the whole leg.*

Effleurage should be performed gently and slowly on individuals who are nervous or who need relaxation. Perform brisk effleurage where stimulation is required (e.g. prior to a sporting activity).

2 Effleuraging the calf

Effleurage the calf muscles only, evenly and rhythmically, but avoid the delicate area at the back of the knee. You are preparing the calf for deeper movements.

3 Dividing the gastrocnemius (belly-shaped muscle)

Position yourself at the receiver's feet.

Starting at the heel use both thumbs to divide the two heads of the gastrocnemius muscle in the calf. Release your pressure just below the back of the knee and glide your hands gently back down to the ankle with no pressure. Repeat this movement several times and feel the muscle fibres separating under your fingers (see Figure 3.2).

4 Petrissage

Now the muscles are warm, position yourself at the side of the receiver's calf to perform the kneading movements. These

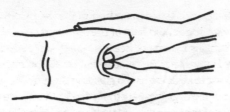

Figure 3.2 *Divide the gastrocnemius muscle of the calf.*

movements will release any toxins that have accumulated in the deeper tissues and the increased blood supply to the area will carry fresh nutrients to the muscles. Regular effleurage and kneading of the leg muscles is also effective in preventing cramp. Petrissage is an excellent way to relieve stiffness especially after exercise.

Petrissage 1 – pick up and squeeze

Place both hands flat on the calf muscles and pick up, squeeze and release the muscles gently (see Figure 3.3). Ensure that you are using the whole of your hands. The receiver will feel an unpleasant 'pinching' sensation if you use only your fingers and thumbs.

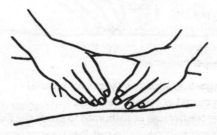

Figure 3.3 *Pick up and squeeze the calf muscles.*

Petrissage 2 – pick up and roll

Squeeze and pick up the calf muscles again and then roll the muscles in both directions. Using your thumbs, roll the muscle towards your fingers and then, using your fingers, roll the muscle towards your thumbs (see Figure 3.4).

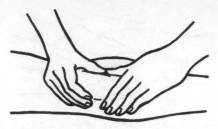

Figure 3.4 *Roll the calf muscles with your thumbs towards your fingers.*

Petrissage 3 – wringing

Place both hands flat on the calf. With alternate hands moving in opposite directions, pick up, squeeze and roll the muscles (see Figure 3.5). Remember as you wring it should look as if you are wringing out a chamois leather.

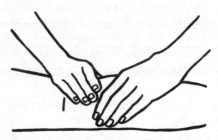

Figure 3.5 *Wring the muscles of the calf.*

5 Completion of lower leg

Effleurage away any toxins that have been released towards the lymph glands in the groin (the inguinal lymph glands).

6 Effleuraging the thigh

Effleurage the whole of the thigh using firm pressure on the way up and no pressure on the return stroke. You are preparing the thigh for deeper massage techniques.

7 Petrissaging the thigh

Wring the inner, middle and outer thigh muscles (see Figure 3.6).

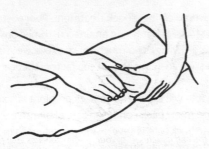

Figure 3.6 *Wring the thigh.*

8 *Percussion movements*

Perform cupping (listen for the hollow sound) and hacking over the whole leg, apart from the back of the knee. These movements will stimulate the circulation and encourage muscle tone. For an even stronger effect you can beat and pound the thighs to help to reduce fatty deposits. Keep your movement light and bouncy!

> Remember!
> * Cupping – palms facing downwards forming a hollow curve.
> * Hacking – palms facing each other, use the edge of the hands.
> * Beating – little finger side of closed fists.
> * Pounding – palmar surface of closed fists.

9 *Completion*

To complete the back of the leg, effleurage the entire leg, gliding your hands back with no pressure. Gradually decrease the pressure with each movement. Rest your cupped hands around the heel to signal that you have finished the posterior leg massage.

Repeat on the other leg.

Back/Shoulders/Neck

Everyone will derive enormous benefits from back massage, irrespective of age. You will be amazed at the number of 'knots' that are discovered during a back treatment. Poor posture, physical or emotional stress, maintaining an unaccustomed position for too long (e.g. gardening), too much sport, excessive studying or a sedentary lifestyle are just some of the factors that can give rise to problems.

Most people will experience a back problem at some time in their life and many back conditions are responsive to massage. However, if the back pain is severe and persistent then always consult a doctor or a fully qualified osteopath as realignment of the vertebrae may be necessary.

Remember not to:
* work on infectious skin conditions
* massage directly over **recent** scar tissue
* work on inflamed or swollen areas
* use friction movements directly over the spine
* use heavy pressure where the skin is thin or bruises easily
* massage over lumps and bumps – check these with a doctor first.

The massage

The receiver should lie in a prone position with one pillow beneath the feet to prevent friction of the toes on the couch, one pillow beneath the head and shoulders and a third pillow under the abdomen if necessary. The receiver will find this position comfortable as it allows all the muscles of the body to relax fully.

If the receiver is pregnant or suffers from a condition that makes lying in the prone position impossible then a side-lying position may be adopted.

The receiver's arms should be at his or her sides or may hang over the edge of the massage couch. The head may be turned to one side or the forehead placed on the hands. The lower half of the body should be covered with a towel and the top towel should be tucked into the underwear.

1 *Effleuraging the entire back*

Position yourself at whichever side of the back you feel most comfortable. Dispense a small amount of oil onto one hand and rub your palms together to warm the oil. Start with both hands in the lower back/buttock area, one hand on either side of the spine, fingers pointing towards the head and effleurage upwards towards the neck. As your hands reach the top of the back spread them outwards across the shoulders (see Figure 3.7). To complete the effleurage movement return to the original position, letting your hands glide back without any pressure. Repeat this movement several times to induce relaxation, to establish your own rhythm and to accustom the receiver to your hands. Close your eyes to heighten sensitivity. Gradually increase your pressure with each movement checking with your partner how much pressure they like.

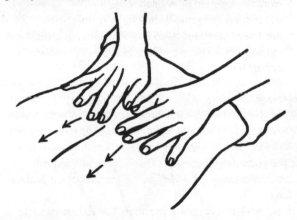

Figure 3.7 *Effleurage the back.*

2 *Lateralizing effleurage to the whole back*

Place your hands down flat on either side of (but not directly on to) the spine with the heels of your hands facing each other, and effleurage outwards (see Figure 3.8). Repeat this movement as necessary, gradually working upwards to cover the entire back. This is a wonderful movement for opening up the back.

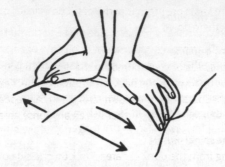

Figure 3.8 *Friction up the back from the base of the spine to the neck.*

3 *Friction to the spinal muscles*

Place the balls of your thumbs in the two dimples that may be visible at the base of the spine and simultaneously friction both sides of the spinal muscles. **Do not** perform these friction movements directly on the spine itself. Proceed up towards the top of the shoulders maintaining the same distance between the thumbs as you travel up the back (see Figure 3.9). Your outward circles should be slow, firm, deep and penetrating as you search out the knots and nodules. If you are performing these movements correctly your thumbs will undoubtedly ache by the time you reach the neck area. Allow your hands to return to the starting point with a feather-light touch. You can friction the spinal muscles several

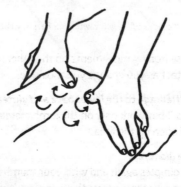

Figure 3.9 *Effleurage outwards across the back.*

times. Where knots are present perform friction circles over them to try to break them down.

4 Spinal thumb gliding

Place the balls of your thumbs in the dimples again and glide your thumbs up towards the neck with firm pressure. Keep your hands in light contact on the return stroke. You can repeat this movement several times to further soften any tense areas.

5 Ironing the spinal muscles

Starting from the buttocks area, work up one side of the back using pushing ironing movements with alternate hands. Follow the movements through with your forearms, working up and over the shoulders and back down again (see Figure 3.10). **Do not work directly over the spine.** This movement not only feels wonderful but releases tension from the muscles and flushes away any toxins released by the friction movements.

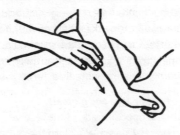

Figure 3.10 *Drain the sides of the back with your hands, wrists and forearms.*

Repeat these ironing movements on the other side of the back. Do not lose contact as you change your position.

6 Lateralizing effleurage to the lower back and gluteals (buttocks)

Repeat step 2 but work only on the lumbar area and buttocks to warm up and open up the area.

7 Frictioning the iliac crest

Locate the dimples again and with your thumbs use deep circular friction movements across the iliac crest (top of the pelvis)

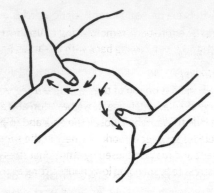

Figure 3.11 *Friction around the iliac crest.*

(see Figure 3.11). This movement breaks up nodules and loosens the pelvis.

8 *Circling the gluteals (buttocks) in a figure of eight*

Place one of your hands flat on the sacrum, and rest the other hand on top of this hand. Using the whole of your hand, circle around the right buttock and back to the sacrum and then over the left buttock returning to the sacrum. Repeat this movement several times.

9 *Petrissaging the lumbar area and gluteals*

Working from the opposite side of the receiver petrissage the gluteals and the lower back area. Work into the muscles slowly and thoroughly as you squeeze, roll and wring the buttocks.

Repeat step 9 on the other side.

Most people have tension in the buttock area. Working in this area not only relieves muscle spasm but also helps break down fatty deposits and helps to tone the area.

10 *Percussion*

Cup and hack the buttock area. You can also beat and pound this region with loosely clenched fists, taking care not to treat any area that is not adequately covered with flesh. These movements will help to break down fatty deposits and induce tone.

11 *Effleurage*

Effleurage the entire back, remembering to use firm pressure on the upward stroke, yet flowing back with a feather-light touch.

12 *Shoulder circling*

Place one hand flat on top of the other and using your whole hand make large circular effleurage movements on and around the shoulder blade to warm and loosen the area and to prepare the shoulder blades for deeper work. Stiffness in the shoulder area is always present and may be caused by emotional stress or by occupational stress (e.g. spending long hours sitting at a desk).

13 *Friction to the scapulae*

The receiver should bend and place the arm behind the back, which will make it easier for you to see the scapula (shoulder blade). Apply deep circular friction movements all round the shoulder blade (see Figure 3.12). As you encounter the knots and nodules, try to remove them with a few friction circles. Always ensure that you are not causing too much discomfort.

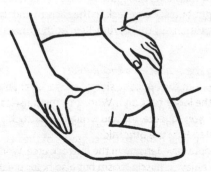

Figure 3.12 *Apply deep friction all around the shoulder blade.*

If the receiver finds it uncomfortable to place the arm behind the back due to tightness in the area then simply leave the arm at the side. Friction around the scapulae will help to improve mobility.

Repeat steps 12 and 13 on the other shoulder blade.

14 *Petrissaging across the shoulders*

Work across the top of the shoulders, rhythmically picking up, squeezing and wringing the trapezius and neighbouring muscles with alternate hands (see Figure 3.13). This movement will loosen the shoulders and relieve any muscular tension.

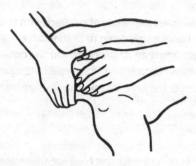

Figure 3.13 *Wring across the top of the shoulders.*

15 *Draining the shoulder region*

To drain any toxins released into the axilla (armpit), effleurage firmly out and down the inside of the scapulae to the axillary lymph nodes in the armpits.

16 *Loosening the neck*

Ask the receiver to place his or her forehead onto their hands in order to straighten the neck. Roll up a small towel and place it under the forehead for extra comfort. Place both your hands flat down, moulding your hands to the contours of the neck. Pick up and squeeze the neck muscles slowly and gently. Ensure that you use the whole of your hands and not just the fingers, which will cause an uncomfortable pinching sensation. The neck is a delicate area requiring great care. It is an important area to massage since tension and stiffness in the neck often gives rise to headaches, migraines and even dizziness.

17 *Effleurage*

Effleurage the entire back.

18 *Feathering the back*

Relax your hands and gently stroke them down either side of the spine using just your fingertips. Repeat this light downwards stroking movement several times. This will completely relax your massage partner.

19 *Completion*

Completely cover the whole of the back with towels and very gently let your hands come down to rest intuitively on the back. Hold your hands lightly on an area that you feel drawn to.

Ask the receiver to turn over. Place a pillow/cushion under the head and one under the knees to take the pressure off the lower back.

Front of the body

Face

The benefits of face massage: Massage treatment of the face is an effective way to relieve headaches of all descriptions, whether caused by stress, sinus congestion, menstrual or digestive problems. As the circulation to the face is improved, the complexion is rejuvenated and takes on a healthy glow. Some individuals opt for regular facial massage in preference to a face lift as the effects are so noticeable. People can look years younger.

Remember not to:
* massage over contact lenses
* work on inflamed or swollen areas
* massage over **recent** scar tissue
* massage over infectious skin conditions or areas of infection such as spots or boils
* use heavy pressure on the face.

The massage

1 *Effleuraging the forehead*

Position yourself at the receiver's head and disperse a small amount of oil onto the palm of one hand and rub your hands together to warm it slightly. Take care not to use too much oil on the face. Stroke out across the forehead using the relaxed fingertips

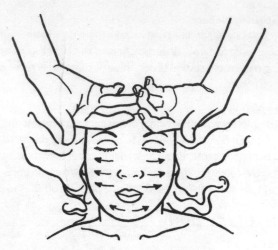

Figure 3.14 *Effleurage the forehead, cheeks and chin.*

of the back of your hands (see Figure 3.14). Let your hands glide back with no pressure.

2 Effleuraging the cheek area

Stroke outwards across the cheeks towards the ears.

3 Effleuraging the chin

Stroke outwards across the chin and jaw and continue to effleurage down the neck towards the armpits to encourage drainage.

4 Decongesting the forehead

Place both thumbs in the centre of the receiver's forehead, just above the eyebrows, with your fingers around the sides of the head. Slowly but firmly press and release at intervals, working outwards in a row. Work up the forehead in strips covering the whole forehead as far as the hairline.

5 Decongesting the cheek area

Start under the eyes, and with your thumbs stroke outwards across the cheeks. Cover the whole of the cheek area in horizontal strips, and as you reach the ears massage them using your thumbs and first two fingers. Stretch and release the ears gently.

6 *Decongesting the chin*

Begin just under the mouth, and with your thumbs press outwards. Cover the entire chin and jaw area, again working in horizontal strips (see Figure 3.15).

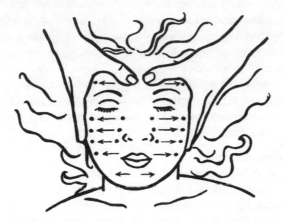

Figure 3.15 *Work across the face in strips using pressure points.*

7 *Unblocking the nasal passages*

Using both thumbs stroke down the sides of the nose.

8 *Releasing the scalp tension*

Using your fingertips, massage the hairline from the top of the forehead around to the base of the skull with deep circular friction movements. Perform these movements firmly and slowly.

9 *Completion*

Stroke the hair gently from the roots to the tips to release the last remaining tension. Gradually allow your hands to come to rest on the temples.

Upper chest and neck

The benefits of chest and neck massage: The chest area plays a vital role in the breathing process. If it is constricted by tension, the ribcage is unable to expand and contract as we breathe in and breathe out. Excessive tightness in the chest can even lead to conditions such as panic attacks, hyperventilation (over-breathing) and other anxiety states where an individual may mistakenly believe that he or she is experiencing a heart attack. Massage of the chest area enables us to breathe more deeply and evenly and also aids the elimination of toxins and mucus. Emotional problems may often be stored in the chest area – in our everyday language we have the expression 'get if off your chest'. Massage encourages us to release these bottled-up emotions.

The neck area is vulnerable to physical and emotional stress and tension. Contraction in the neck muscles is a major contributory factor to headaches. Massage is an excellent way of relieving this tension.

Remember not to:
* apply heavy pressure to the chest and neck
* massage inflamed or sensitive areas
* massage infectious skin conditions
* work directly over **recent** scar tissue, open wounds or recent fractures
* massage over lumps: these should be checked by a doctor.

The massage

1 *Effleuraging the chest*

Position yourself at the receiver's head and place your hands in the centre of the chest just below the clavicles (collarbones). Relax your fingers and, with the back of both hands, effleurage gently outwards towards the armpits (see Figure 3.16). As you reach the shoulders, turn your hands over and use the palms to stroke and direct the lymph into the axillary glands under the arms. Stroke back with no pressure to the starting position. Repeat several

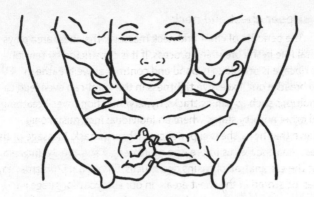

Figure 3.16 *Effleurage across the upper chest.*

times. Effleurage warms up the chest, prepares the chest for deeper movements and encourages the elimination of toxins.

2 Frictioning the chest

Start in the centre of the receiver's chest below the clavicles. Make gentle circular friction movements with your thumbs or fingers, working towards and around the front of the shoulders.

3 Knuckling the chest

Make both hands into loose fists and make gentle circular movements over the upper chest area. These movements on the pectoral muscles help to release further tension in the chest.

4 Stretching the chest and shoulder muscles

Cup your hands around the top of both shoulders and gently push the shoulders down towards the feet. Repeat several times.

Move your hands so that they cup the front of the shoulders, and with straight arms, press down. Hold this position for approximately five seconds and release slowly. Repeat several times to loosen up the shoulder girdle.

5 Releasing the neck

Reach under the neck with both hands so that your fingertips touch and gently stroke, pulling up and towards you. This will allow any muscular tension to dissolve.

6 *Side stroking*

Turn the head to one side. Place one hand on the forehead and stroke the other hand from the ear, down the side of the neck and over the shoulder. Repeat on the other side of the neck. Stroking the neck releases tension, drains toxins and gently stretches the neck.

7 *Frictioning around the base of the skull*

With the head straight, feel the base of the skull with the fingers of both hands. Make circular friction movements around the base of the skull to release any nodules. Many headaches arise due to tightness at the base of the skull.

8 *Stretching the neck*

Cup both your hands under the back of the head, with the fingers at the base of the skull. Pull gently and slowly towards you as you lean backwards, thus using your own body weight to traction the neck. Never jerk or pull the neck suddenly.

9 *Completion*

Rest your cupped hands gently on the forehead to relax and soothe the receiver.

Arm and hand

The benefits of arm and hand massage: Our arms and hands are in constant use in our everyday activities in the home, at work and in our leisure pursuits. It is not surprising that they are prone to so many injuries. Massage can afford a great deal of relief.

Remember not to:
* work over recent fractures
* massage directly over areas of inflammation such as swollen joints
* massage directly over **recent** scar tissue
* massage infectious skin conditions
* use heavy pressure where the skin is thin or bruises easily
* use heavy pressure on the delicate area at the front of the elbow joint.

The massage

1 *Effleuraging the arm*

Position yourself at the side of the arm to be treated and effleurage the entire arm from the wrist to the shoulder. You may perform this effleurage in two ways:

1. Support the arm carefully underneath with one hand as you effleurage (if necessary you may use a pillow too).
2. Use one hand to 'shake hands' with the receiver and the other to effleurage.

Stroking the arms improves the circulation, aids drainage and prepares the arm for deeper movements. The arm is elevated whilst effleuraging to ensure maximum drainage.

2 *Frictioning the shoulder*

To loosen and mobilize the shoulder joint use slow circular friction movements around the front, top and back of the shoulder joint.

3 *Petrissaging the upper arm*

Bend the receiver's arm and place the forearm across the body so that it is resting and supported on the receiver's upper abdomen. Pick up, roll and wring the biceps and triceps muscles of the upper arm firmly and rhythmically. Petrissaging the arm will relieve muscular tension, bring toxins to the surface and help to break down fatty deposits.

4 *Frictioning the elbow*

Whilst supporting the arm, use the circular friction movements around the elbow joint to relieve pain and stiffness. If there is any sensitivity then decrease your pressure circles.

5 *Effleuraging the arm*

Effleurage the entire arm to encourage any toxins that have been released to move towards the axillary lymph glands in the armpit.

6 *Effleuraging the forearm*

With the receiver's upper arm down and the forearm lifted, effleurage firmly from the wrist to the elbow (see Figure 3.17).

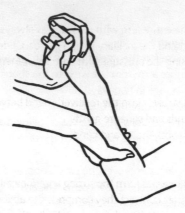

Figure 3.17 *Effleurage the forearm from wrist to elbow.*

7 Frictioning the wrist joint

Using your thumbs, friction into the bones of the wrist to loosen it.

8 Mobilizing the wrist

Interlock your fingers with the receiver's fingers (if the size of the hands are compatible) and bend the wrist slowly, gently and carefully backwards and forwards, side to side and circumduct the wrist clockwise and anticlockwise. This is excellent exercise for improving mobility in the wrist.

9 Frictioning the hand

Friction with your thumbs into the palm of the receiver's hand and also into the back of the hand. This will loosen the joints, muscles and tendons of the hand.

10 Mobilizing the fingers

To work the 14 phalanges (finger joints and thumb joints), gently and slowly squeeze and stretch each finger individually. With your thumb and index finger friction the phalanges. Flex and extend each phalange – there are two in the thumb joint and three in the fingers. Circumduct each finger individually clockwise and anticlockwise.

11 *Effleurage*

Effleurage the entire arm with pressure, as always, up the arm towards the heart and the axilliary lymph glands. Glide gently back, gradually decreasing the pressure with each movement.

12 *Completion*

On the final stroke, clasp the receiver's hand between the palms of your hands and squeeze gently.

Repeat on the other arm and hand.

Abdomen

Four pairs of muscles form the strong anterior wall of the abdomen. When they contract they compress the abdomen – thus they help in functions such as defecation, childbirth, forced expiration and so on. They also have a very important postural function in that they pull the front of the pelvis upwards, flattening the lumbar curve of the spine. If these muscles lose their tone then the abdomen protrudes.

The abdomen is an often neglected area of the body as far as massage is concerned. Remember when massaging the abdomen that you are working on muscles and organs. The benefits that can be derived from abdominal massage are considerable.

The benefits of abdominal massage include:

* Constipation, bloatedness and flatulence can be relieved. If the problem is chronic then diet and nutrition should be altered.
* After an operation (e.g. Caesarean or appendix), once scar tissue has begun to heal, massage will help to prevent adhesion formation and scar contractures.
* If there is visceroptosis (prolapse of the viscera) where the contents of the abdomen drop to a lower level, massage will help if it is combined with exercise, provided that there is still some tone left in the muscles. If muscle tone is restored to the outer wall by massage then the internal organs may be held in a normal position. Visceroptosis may occur due to incorrect posture, abdominal surgery, inadequate support or insufficient muscle toning after childbirth.

Remember not to:

* massage over **recent** scar tissue until it has healed and only then with the permission of a doctor (once healing is established massage is excellent for preventing adhesions).
* massage where there is inflammation of any organs in the abdomen (e.g. gastritis, appendicitis, colitis)
* massage the abdomen within one hour of a heavy meal
* use heavy pressure over the abdomen during pregnancy
* use heavy pressure during the first few days of menstruation if it is uncomfortable
* encourage the receiver to talk or laugh during the abdominal massage because the muscles tighten making treatment impossible
* massage the abdomen if the bladder is full (suggest a visit to the lavatory prior to a treatment).

The massage

1 *Circular effleurage (two handed)*

Make sure you are positioned on the receiver's right-hand side when you start the massage so that you are able to follow the colon in the appropriate direction. Place both your hands on the receiver's navel, one hand on top of the other, and move in a clockwise direction with a circular movement (see Figure 3.18). Gradually increase the size of the circles until the entire abdomen is covered. Use gentle pressure at first, gradually increasing the depth of the strokes as the receiver relaxes.

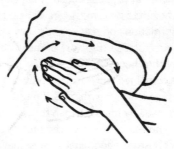

Figure 3.18 *Double-handed effleurage of the abdomen.*

2 Circular effleurage (one handed)

Moving in a clockwise direction, circle around the abdomen with one hand following behind the other (see Figure 3.19).

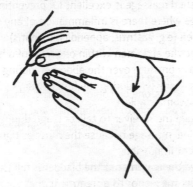

Figure 3.19 *Circular effleurage of the abdomen, one hand following the other.*

3 Colon massage

To treat the colon, begin at the bottom right-hand side of the abdomen. With the flat surface of the three middle fingers of one hand work around the colon in a clockwise direction using small circular friction movements (see Figure 3.20).

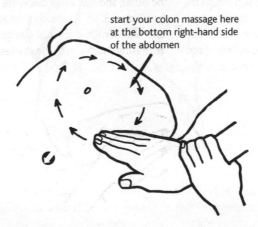

start your colon massage here at the bottom right-hand side of the abdomen

Figure 3.20 *Gently massage the colon.*

Slide your hand across the abdomen to the starting position using no pressure. Repeat several times to help relieve digestive problems such as constipation.

4 Circular effleurage

Repeat the clockwise circular stroking, working smoothly with one hand following the other to further assist detoxification.

5 Draining the abdomen (one side)

Using both hands, one on top of the other, reach across to the receiver's far side underneath the abdomen and pull upwards and then downwards towards the bladder. Repeat on the other side of the abdomen.

6 Draining the abdomen (both sides)

Reach under the receiver's abdomen so that your fingers are touching each other (waistline permitting). Pull both hands at the same time upwards and downwards towards the bladder (see Figure 3.21). Draining the abdomen reduces bloating and fluid retention.

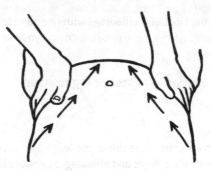

Figure 3.21 *Drain the abdomen.*

7 Petrissaging

Pick up and roll and wring the waist and hip area opposite you. Repeat on the other side of the waist and hip area. Petrissage will help to improve the tone of the abdomen.

8 *Gentle percussion*

Reaching over the opposite side, **gently** cup and hack the waist and hip area to increase muscular tone and to break down fatty deposits.

9 *Circular effleurage*

Effleurage the entire abdomen with one hand following the other.

10 *Rocking the pelvis*

Using your palms, place one hand on each side of the receiver's pelvis. Rock gently and slowly. This movement loosens the pelvic area and encourages the whole body to relax.

11 *Vibration of the abdomen*

Gently place both hands, one on top of the other, on the abdomen and then vibrate your hands rapidly yet gently up and down or from side to side. Vibration of the abdomen aids digestion and relieves flatulence and constipation.

12 *Completion*

Repeat the clockwise effleurage with one hand following the other. Gradually decrease the pressure and let your hands come to rest on the navel.

Front of the leg (anterior leg massage)

The massage

1 *Effleuraging the leg*

Position yourself at the side of the leg to be massaged. Warm the oil between your hands and effleurage the entire leg from the ankle to the top of the thigh, using only light pressure over the knee. Mould your hands to the contours of the leg. Cup your hands over the front of the ankle, one hand above the other and, as you reach the top of the thigh, separate your hands and glide them gently down the sides of the leg. These movements stimulate the circulation and eliminate toxins.

2 *Effleuraging the thigh*

Firmly effleurage the whole of the thigh – pressure on the way up, feather-light touch on the return.

3 *Petrissaging the thigh*

Pick up, roll and wring the inner, middle and outer thigh muscles to bring the deeper toxins to the surface and to eliminate fatty deposits and release muscular tension.

4 *Effleuraging the thigh*

Effleurage the thigh to eliminate further toxins.

5 *Patella*

Work all around the patella (kneecap) using small circular friction movements (see Figure 3.22). Notice how small the kneecap is. Friction movements will help to give more mobility to the knee joint.

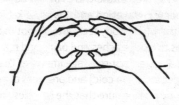

Figure 3.22 *Use small circular movements around the patella (kneecap).*

6 *Effleuraging the lower leg*

Effleurage the lower half of the leg with cupped hands from ankle to knee. Use less pressure on this bony, more delicate area than you did on the thigh.

7 *Gentle friction on the lower leg*

Gently friction along the outside of the tibialis anterior muscle of the lower leg. You can see this muscle easily if the receiver pulls his or her foot up.

8 *Effleurage*

Effleurage the entire leg.

9 *Percussion*

Cup and hack the thigh only. For a stronger effect use beating and pounding too. Never perform percussion movements over the bony areas of the lower leg. Percussion movements stimulate circulation and reduce fatty deposits and cellulite and tone the muscles.

10 *Completion*

Effleurage the entire leg, gradually decreasing the pressure with each movement.

Repeat on the other leg.

Foot

The benefits of foot massage: Our feet have to support the weight of our entire body and they also act as shock absorbers – no wonder they feel so tired at the end of a hard day! Massage of the feet is marvellous for relaxation and it is remarkable how refreshed and revitalized the whole body feels after a foot massage. Treatment of the feet helps to relieve aches and pains and maintains flexibility and suppleness. Regular foot massage improves the circulation dramatically (feet are often cold) and prevents cramp in the sole of the foot by making sure that the muscles are cleansed of toxins.

Remember not to:

* use heavy pressure on varicose veins or where a person has thin skin and/or bruises easily (e.g. a person with diabetes)
* massage over **recent** scar tissue or painful areas
* massage directly over contagious skin conditions – for example athlete's foot, verrucae
* massage firmly over corns or blisters if it causes pain
* use too much oil as this will make some of the movements impossible to perform.

The massage

1 *Effleuraging the foot*

Effleurage the whole foot **firmly** using both hands to avoid tickling. Cover the dorsum (top) of the foot, the sides of the foot and the plantar aspect (sole) of the foot. Work from the ends of the toes to the top of the foot (see Figure 3.23). Slide around the ankle bones and glide back. Effleuraging the foot improves circulation and prepares the foot for deeper work.

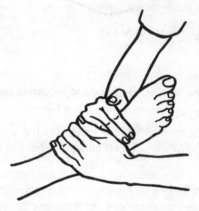

Figure 3.23 *Effleurage the foot.*

2 *Frictioning the sole of the foot*

With one hand supporting the heel, friction the entire sole of the foot (see Figure 3.24). Begin underneath the big toe and work outwards towards the little toe. Continue to friction the remainder of the plantar aspect (sole) of the foot in horizontal strips until you have covered the whole area. These movements loosen muscles and tendons.

3 *Effleurage*

Effleurage the foot to eliminate any waste products you have released.

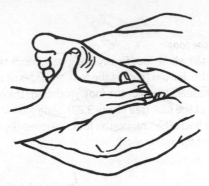

Figure 3.24 *Friction the sole of the foot.*

4 *Frictioning the toes*
Friction the toe joints both top and bottom to loosen them.

5 *Mobilizing the toes*
Supporting the heel with one hand, stretch and circumduct each toe individually. This will encourage flexibility of the toes.

6 *Effleurage*
Effleurage the foot.

7 *Frictioning the ankle*
Friction around the ankle joint using both thumbs to loosen it.

8 *Mobilizing the ankle*
Supporting the foot with one hand, slowly but firmly dorsiflex the foot (push it backwards) and plantarflex the foot (point it). Now invert (turn the sole inwards) and evert (turn the sole outwards) the foot. Then circumduct the foot clockwise and anticlockwise. Notice how the mobility of the ankle improves.

9 *Vibrations*
Place the palms of your hands one on each side of the foot, and move them alternately and rapidly side to side so that the foot vibrates (see Figure 3.25).

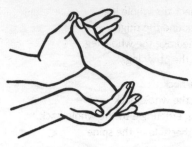

Figure 3.25 *Move the foot rapidly from side to side.*

10 *Completion*

Effleurage the foot gently, and to complete the foot massage clasp the foot between both of your hands and squeeze gently.

Repeat on the other foot.

Well done! You have completed a full body massage.

At the end of the treatment wash your hands thoroughly under cold, running water to cleanse yourself physically and psychically.

Massage sequence memory jogger

Back of the body

Back of the legs

1 Effleurage the whole leg (v-shape)
2 Effleurage the calf
3 Divide the calf muscle
4 Petrissage the calf:
   * Pick up, squeeze and release
   * Pick up and roll (both directions)
   * Wring
5 Effleurage the whole leg
6 Firmly effleurage the thigh
7 Wring the inner, middle and outer thigh

8 Cup and hack the whole leg
   9 Beat and pound the thigh
  10 Gently effleurage the whole leg.
     Repeat on the other leg.

Back/shoulders/neck

   1 Effleurage the whole back
   2 Lateralizing effleurage to the whole back
   3 Friction either side of the spine
   4 Spinal thumb gliding
   5 Iron the spinal muscles
   6 Lateralizing effleurage to the lower back and buttocks
   7 Friction across the iliac crest (top of the pelvis)
   8 Figure of eight circling over the buttocks
   9 Petrissage the lower back area and buttocks
  10 Percussion on the buttocks area (cup, hack, beat and
     pound)
  11 Effleurage the whole back
  12 Circular effleurage on the shoulder blade
  13 Friction around the shoulder blade
     Repeat steps 12 and 13 on the other shoulder blade.
  14 Petrissage across the shoulders
  15 Effleurage towards the armpits to drain
  16 Pick up and squeeze the neck
  17 Effleurage the whole back
  18 Feather the back.

Front of the body

Face

   1 Effleurage the forehead, cheeks and chin
   2 Decongest the forehead, cheeks and chin (press and release in
     horizontal strips)
   3 Stroke down the sides of the nose
   4 Friction the scalp
   5 Stroke the hair.

Upper chest and neck

1 Effleurage across the chest towards the armpits
2 Gentle friction across the chest just below the collarbones
3 Knuckle the chest
4 Push down the shoulders
5 Stroke up the neck
6 Stroke down the sides of the neck
7 Friction around the base of the skull
8 Stretch the neck
9 Rest your hands gently on the forehead.

Arm and hand

1 Effleurage the whole arm
2 Friction around the shoulder joint
3 Petrissage the upper arm
4 Friction around the elbow
5 Effleurage the whole arm
6 Effleurage the forearm
7 Friction around the wrist joint
8 Interlock the fingers to carefully move the wrist backwards and forwards, side to side, clockwise and anticlockwise
9 Friction into the palm of the hand
10 Slowly squeeze and stretch each finger individually, mobilize each finger joint, circumduct each finger clockwise and anticlockwise
11 Effleurage the whole arm.
12 Gently squeeze the receiver's hand.
Repeat on the other arm and hand.

Abdomen

N.B. Position yourself on the right-hand side of the abdomen
1 Circular effleurage in a clockwise direction one hand on top of the other
2 Circular effleurage one hand following the other
3 Gentle colon friction with fingertips
4 Circular effleurage

5 Drain the sides of the abdomen
6 Petrissage the waist and hip area
7 Gently cup and hack the waist and hip area
8 Circular effleurage
9 Rock the pelvis
10 Vibration on the abdomen
11 Circular effleurage.

Front of the leg

1 Effleurage the whole leg
2 Effleurage the thigh
3 Petrissage the thigh
4 Effleurage the thigh
5 Friction all around the patella (kneecap)
6 Effleurage the lower leg
7 Gentle friction along the outside of the lower leg
8 Effleurage the whole leg
9 Percussion on the thigh only (cup, hack, beat, pound)
10 Effleurage the whole leg.
   Repeat on the other leg.

Foot

1 Effleurage the foot
2 Friction the sole of the foot
3 Effleurage the foot
4 Friction the toe joints
5 Stretch and circumduct each toe individually
6 Effleurage the foot
7 Friction around the ankle to loosen it and then slowly move
   the ankle in all directions
8 Move the foot rapidly from side to side
9 Effleurage the foot gently.
   Repeat on the other foot.

4

self-massage

It is easily possible, and very pleasurable, to massage your own legs, feet, neck and shoulders, back, abdomen, arms and hands, and face and scalp for optimum health.

Self-massage has the advantage that you can perform it as often as you wish at almost any time and place. It is a wonderful way to soothe away your stress and tension and to treat many common disorders such as aching, tired legs and feet, back pain, stiff neck, colon problems (such as constipation) and headaches.

As you massage yourself, notice which movements feel particularly good. The more you practise on yourself, the more proficient you will become at massaging your friends and family. An added bonus is that you will feel more relaxed and full of vitality.

Ideally you should massage yourself at least once a week. If you are experiencing discomfort such as low back pain or a sore neck then massage the affected area daily. You will be amazed at the relief.

Legs

Massage will help to relieve your tired and achy legs at the end of the day. You can prevent varicose veins, improve circulation, reduce swelling and improve the appearance of unsightly cellulite.

A simple leg massage prior to or after exercise is a wonderful way of preventing injuries and relieving stiffness.

Position for massage

Sit down on the floor or on a bed with one leg stretched out straight in front of you and the other leg bent with the foot flat on the ground.

1 *Calf muscles – effleurage*

Effleurage from your heel to the back of your knee using one or both hands (see Figure 4.1). Place both hands at the front of the leg and stroke upwards.

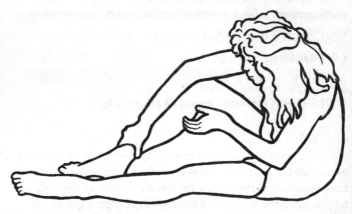

Figure 4.1 *Effleurage the calf.*

2 Calf muscles – petrissage

Keeping your knee bent, work on your calf muscles at the back of your leg. Pick up, roll and wring this area. This is an excellent way to prevent and relieve cramps and muscle spasm.

3 Achilles tendon – friction

With your fingers and thumbs apply deep friction to your Achilles tendon.

4 Knee – friction

Place the pads of both thumbs just below the knee and use small circular friction movements all around the patella. These movements will help to improve and maintain mobility of your knee joint.

5 Thigh – effleurage

Stroke firmly up from the knee towards the groin. Ensure that you effleurage all aspects of the thigh.

6 Thigh – petrissage

Squeeze and wring the inner, middle and outer thigh muscles. This can help to break down fatty deposits and if performed daily may greatly improve the shape of your thighs! If you wish to pay extra attention to certain areas then make your hands into loose fists and perform circular movements with your knuckles.

7 Cellulite buster!

Lightly clench your fists and bring them down onto any areas of cellulite in quick succession.

Finish with effleurage. Repeat on the other leg.

Feet

Massage of the feet is not only a very pleasurable and relaxing experience but it also helps to improve the health of the entire body. According to reflexology, the feet are a mirror of the body and by massaging the feet you are treating all the organs, glands and structures of the body.

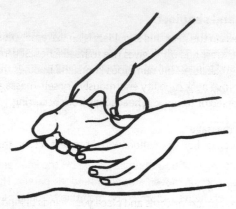

Figure 4.2 *Friction the sole.*

Position for massage

Sit down on the floor, on a bed or a chair. Bend the knee and place the foot to be treated on the opposite thigh (see Figure 4.2).

1 *Foot – effleurage*

With one hand under the sole of the foot and the other on the top, stroke firmly upwards.

2 *Foot – friction the sole*

Use both thumbs to make small circular movements all over the sole of the foot. This opens up and loosens the tendons and muscles of the foot.

3 *Ankle – friction and move*

Use your thumbs or fingertips to make circular movements all around the ankle joint. Gently and slowly circle your ankle both clockwise and anticlockwise.

4 *Toes – friction and move*

Using your thumb and index finger, friction the toe joints both top and bottom to loosen them. Then slowly stretch and move each of them both clockwise and anticlockwise.

Finish with effleurage and repeat on the other foot.

Neck and shoulders

Tightness in the neck and shoulders is an extremely common symptom of stress and often gives rise to headaches. Self-massage can help to break down the numerous knots and nodules that arise and will improve neck mobility enormously. Try self-massage when you feel stressed or to prevent headaches from occurring.

Position for massage

Sit on a chair, bed or the floor with both feet flat on the ground.

1 *Neck – effleurage*

Relax your neck forwards and place your hands behind your head, fingertips touching or slightly overlapping. Apply deep, downwards effleurage movements down the neck.

2 *Neck – friction*

Apply small circular friction movements to the base of your skull using your fingertips to prevent headaches from occurring.

3 *Shoulders – effleurage*

To massage your right shoulder reach across the front of your chest and place your left hand at the base of the skull and stroke firmly down the side of the neck and over your shoulder.

4 *Shoulders – pick up and squeeze*

Reach across the front of your chest again and slowly squeeze and release the muscles on top of the other shoulder picking up as much flesh as possible.

Repeat steps 3 and 4 on the other shoulder.

5 *Scapulae – friction*

Reach across the front of your body with your right hand to touch your left shoulder blade at the back of your body (See Figure 4.3). Use your fingertips to apply deep pressure to any knots or nodules.

Repeat on the other shoulder blade.

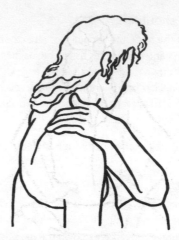

Figure 4.3 *Friction of the scapula (shoulder blade).*

Back

Most of you will suffer from back pain at least once in your lifetime. Self-massage of the back can dramatically reduce back pain. If you are prone to back problems perform this routine daily.

The back is a difficult area to reach without stretching, but it is worth persevering for the benefits you will derive.

Position for massage

Sit down on the floor, on a stool or on a bed.

1 Back – friction

Press your thumbs into the dimples on either side of your spine. Perform circular friction movements working up your back slowly and deeply, travelling as far up as you can (see Figure 4.4). Search out the knots and nodules and when you encounter them apply firmer pressure to break them down. If you find it difficult to use your thumbs then use the pads of several of your fingers instead.

2 Back – effleurage

Place your hands behind your back, one flat palm either side of your spine. Firmly effleurage down your back. Perform this

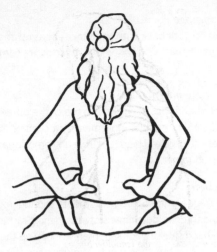

Figure 4.4 *Friction the back.*

movement slowly to relax and soothe or quickly to stimulate and invigorate. This movement may also be performed using lightly clenched fists.

3 Back – circular effleurage

Place both hands in the middle of your lower back, fingertips pointing downwards. Make large outward circles with both hands simultaneously to loosen and decongest the lumbar area and buttocks. If you need a deeper treatment, use the knuckles of your fists.

Abdomen

Abdominal massage will encourage regular bowel movements, relieve the discomfort of abdominal bloating and aid the digestion, absorption and elimination of food. After abdominal surgery such as a Caesarean or an appendicectomy, once the scar tissue has healed, massage helps to prevent the formation of adhesions and speeds up recovery. If performed daily, muscle tone will also be improved.

Position for massage

Lie down on your back with your knees bent up and your feet apart so that your abdominal muscles are completely relaxed.

1 *Abdomen – circular effleurage*

Place your hands flat down, one on top of the other on your navel. Make large slow circular movements, proceeding in a clockwise direction. These strokes will help to relieve any emotional trauma stored in your abdomen.

2 *Colon – friction*

To encourage regular bowel movements, friction your colon gently with the three middle fingers of your hand. Start at the bottom right-hand side of your abdomen working up the ascending colon. Friction across the abdomen to stimulate the transverse colon. To complete your colon massage, work down the descending colon to the left-hand side of your abdomen.

3 *Abdomen – gentle percussion*

To stimulate digestion and improve muscle tone, perform very gentle cupping.

Arm and hand

Our arms, wrists and hands are used constantly in our daily activities. Aches and pains in the arms and hands are often caused by repetitive movements, although they may be the result of a neck problem. Massage of these areas is essential to promote strength and mobility and is particularly beneficial to people who use their hands and arms extensively in the course of their work – for example individuals who use computer keyboards, gardeners and hairdressers. Treatment is also essential for sports people for preventing injuries from occurring. According to hand reflexology all the parts of the body are mirrored in miniature on the hands.

Position for massage

Sit down on the floor, bed or a chair. Rest one hand gently on your lap.

1 Arm – effleurage

Place the palm of your hand on your wrist and effleurage the whole arm up to the shoulder.

2 Upper arm – effleurage

Apply deep stroking to the flexor muscles on the front of your upper arm (biceps, brachialis) and the extensor muscles (triceps) on the back of your upper arm. Always work up your arm trying to move the lymph up towards the axillary glands in your armpit.

3 Upper arm – petrissage

Pick up and squeeze and wring the muscles of your upper arm to break down any adhesions and to bring the deeper toxins to the surface.

4 Lower arm – deep stroking

With your elbow flexed and the tip of your elbow resting on your abdomen to encourage drainage, apply deep downward longitudinal stroking to the flexor and extensor muscles of your lower arm.

5 Wrist – loosen and move

Use your thumb and fingertips to gently friction all around the wrist joint. After these loosening movements interlock your fingers and circle the wrist clockwise and anticlockwise.

6 Palm – circular kneading

With a clenched fist, work into the palm of your hand with circular movements to loosen up the muscles, tendons and joints.

7 Fingers and thumb – loosen and move

Using your thumb and index finger gently stretch each finger and thumb. Then circle each one individually. These movements will ease rheumatic complaints and arthritis.

Repeat on the other arm and hand.

Face and scalp

Face and scalp massage is a wonderful way to relax and unwind, completely banishing tiredness and anxiety, relieving headaches and clearing sinuses. Over a period of time, as circulation and drainage is stimulated, you will also notice improvements in your complexion and fine wrinkles may disappear.

Position for massage

Lie down on the floor or bed, or sit up on a chair if you prefer.

1 *Face – effleurage*

Place both hands palms down on your forehead with your fingertips facing each other. Stroke across your forehead. Repeat this outward movement, stroking across your cheeks and across your chin.

2 *Eyes – stroking*

Use your index or your index and middle fingers to effleurage very gently outwards underneath each eye. Take great care, as this is a very delicate area. These movements will help to relieve puffiness and to prevent and reduce fine lines.

3 *Chin and jaw – toning*

Pinch all along your jaw line using your thumbs and index finger to help prevent a double chin.

4 *Eyebrows – toning*

Starting at the inside of your eyebrows, pinch your brow bone until you reach the end of your eyebrow. Repeat each movement several times.

5 *Mouth – friction*

Make a large 'O' with your mouth. Using your index and middle fingers apply small circular friction movements around your mouth. These movements may help to stop fine wrinkles appearing.

6 *Scalp – friction*

With your fingertips, use small rotary movements covering your entire scalp. These movements will remove tension from your scalp and by aiding circulation can also make your hair healthier.

7 Completion

To finish your massage programme, place the heels of your hands over your eyes. Hold your hands there for a few seconds allowing your eyes to relax completely in darkness as you gently remove your hands. You will feel revitalized and refreshed.

aromatherapy and massage

Using aromatherapy blends with essential oils tailored to your specific requirements can enhance the effects of your massage.

Massage with essential oils is very healing on all levels: it encourages physical, mental, emotional and even spiritual health equilibrium. Frankincense, for example, is excellent on a physical level for all respiratory disorders such as chesty coughs and asthma. On an emotional level it reduces stress and anxiety, calming the emotions and allowing past traumas to fade away so that we can move on. On a spiritual level frankincense enables us to reach a deep meditative state. There is nothing to beat working with the wonderful aromas of essential oils as you impart their therapeutic effects through the magic of massage!

Essential oils

Blending

Essential oils are extremely concentrated. Always blend them with a suitable carrier oil in the appropriate dilution when using them for massage. Lavender and tea tree may be used undiluted to treat injuries such as wasp stings, cuts or burns.

The essential oil content in a blend should usually be between one per cent and three per cent. Use the following as a rough guideline:
* 5 ml carrier oil = 1 teaspoon
* 10 ml carrier oil = 1 dessertspoon
* 15 ml carrier oil = 1 tablespoon
* Add 3 drops of pure essential oil to 10 ml of carrier oil
* Add 5 drops of pure essential oil to 15 ml of carrier oil
* Add 6 drops of pure essential oil to 20 ml of carrier oil.

Storage of essential oils

Essential oils should always be stored in dark coloured rather than clear glass bottles as the oils deteriorate in sunlight. Amber coloured bottles are by far the best. Essential oils are volatile, so replace the caps immediately after use, otherwise the oils will gradually evaporate. Always keep essential oils at an even temperature – avoid direct sunlight and shelves on radiators.

If you keep pure essential oils in amber glass bottles in a cool place, they should have a shelf life of approximately two to three years. Citrus essential oils have the shortest shelf life. Once an essential oil has been diluted in a carrier oil or cream, it will keep for only a few months.

Purchasing

It is important to buy only pure essential oils if you want to achieve the best results. Synthetic and adulterated oils carry with them the risk of unpleasant and harmful side effects. Essential oils may be adulterated by adding alcohol, synthetic products or cheaper essential oils. Make sure you buy pure essential oils, not oils that have already been diluted in a carrier oil.

Massage with essential oils

Massage with essential oils is an extremely powerful method of application. The minute molecules of essential oil penetrate the skin and can reach the bloodstream and lymph. Aromatherapy massage is the only treatment technique discussed in this book. Other methods include inhalations, baths, foot and hand baths, showers, compresses, gargles and mouthwashes. For further information please refer to *Flash: Natural Healing with Aromatherapy*.

I have chosen 16 of the most common essential oils used in aromatherapy today with particular emphasis on their uses and indications. If medical conditions are severe and persistent, consult a qualified medical practitioner before treatment.

Bergamot

Latin name:	*Citrus bergamia*
Family:	RUTACEAE
Keywords:	antidepressant, antiseptic, balancing, uplifting

Principal properties and effects

* An invaluable oil for stress, anxiety and depression, possessing an uplifting yet sedative quality.

* Helpful for infections of the urinary tract, vaginal infections, itching and thrush.
* Beneficial for the digestive system. Relieves indigestion, flatulence and loss of appetite as in anorexia.
* Excellent for infections of the respiratory system including sore throats, tonsillitis and bronchitis.
* Useful for the skin as an antiseptic for acne, seborrhea of the skin and scalp. Also for infectious conditions such as chicken pox and shingles.

If like me you are a fan of Earl Grey tea you will recognize the aroma of bergamot as the leaves of the plant are used in the manufacture of the tea.

Special precautions

Avoid strong sunlight after use as bergamot increases the photosensitivity of the skin due to the chemical bergapten.

Chamomile (Roman)

Latin name:	***Anthemis nobilis***
Family:	**COMPOSITAE/ASTERACEAE**
Keywords:	**balancing, soothing, anti-inflammatory, redness and irritation**

Principal properties and effects

* Excellent for inflammatory disorders such as colitis, gastritis and dermatitis.
* Beneficial for skin care, soothing allergic and hypersensitive skin, boils, burns and inflamed wounds. Helpful for eczema and dry itchy skin.
* Its analgesic action relieves aches and pains whether in muscles, joints or organs – backache, earache, headache, stomach ache, toothache.

* Renowned for its soothing effects on the nervous system, promoting relaxation and deep sleep (chamomile tea is a popular infusion for relieving insomnia). Dispels anger, anxiety, fear and tension.
* Popular for menstrual disorders – painful menstruation, menopause, heavy periods, pre-menstrual syndrome. It balances the hormones, eases period pain, regulates the menstrual cycle and relieves anger and irritability.
* Useful for boosting the immune system. It stimulates the leucocytes (white blood cells) and thus reduces the frequency and severity of infections.

A must have for babies and children, Roman chamomile eases asthma, colic, infections, skin problems and temper tantrums.

Special precautions

None! Roman chamomile is an extremely safe oil.

Cypress

Latin name: *Cupressus sempervirens*
Family: CUPRESSACEAE
Keywords: astringent, fluid reducing, restorative

Principal properties and effects

* Helpful whenever there is excessive fluid – oedema, sweating (particularly of the feet), bedwetting.
* Renowned for regulating the menstrual cycle and for relieving menstrual problems, particularly PMS (pre-menstrual syndrome) and the hot flushes, hormonal imbalances, irritability and depression of the menopause.
* Balances oily skin, puffiness, cellulite.

* Its comforting and restorative properties help to ease grief. Cypress alleviates nervous tension and stress-related conditions.
* Excellent for varicose veins due to its vasoconstricting effect. Use gentle effleurage only.

Cypress is excellent for varicose veins due to its vasoconstricting effect. Blend 2 drops of cypress and one drop of lemon in a carrier oil. Use gentle effleurage working up the legs on a daily basis.

Special precautions

None! Cypress is non-irritant, non-sensitizing and non-toxic.

Eucalyptus

Latin name: *Eucalyptus globulus*
Family: MYRTACEAE
Keywords: analgesic (pain relieving), antiseptic, expectorant (clears out mucus), stimulant

Principal properties and effects

* Invaluable for respiratory disorders.
* Provides pain relief for arthritis, muscular aches and pains and rheumatism.
* Powerful essential oil for stimulating the brain and aiding concentration.
* Effective for all types of fever and infectious illnesses.

Eucalyptus is excellent as a chest rub for all respiratory disorders – asthma, catarrh, colds, coughs, sinusitis and throat infections. For problems affecting the lungs I also recommend working on the back. Remember that cupping when performed over the upper and middle back area loosens mucus in the lungs.

Special precautions

* Store away from homoeopathic medications.
* Do not use on babies and young children.

Frankincense

Latin name: *Boswellia carterii*
Family: BURSERACEAE
Keywords: expectorant, elevating, healing, rejuvenating

Principal properties and effects

* Encourages the breath to slow down and deepen, making it ideal for asthma and all respiratory disorders especially when linked with stress. Particularly conducive to prayer and meditation.
* An excellent remedy for all skin care. Frankincense rejuvenates mature and ageing skin, toning and smoothing out the wrinkles. Heals ulcers and wounds.

Frankincense engenders an elevating yet soothing effect on the emotions allowing past traumas and anxiety to fade away. It helps us to let go and move on.

Special precautions
None.

Geranium

Latin name: *Pelargonium graveolens*
Family: GERANIACEAE
Keywords: antidepressant, balancing, healing, uplifting

Principal properties and effects

* Particularly beneficial for the nervous system, dispelling anxiety states and depression and uplifting the spirit.
* Stimulates the lymphatic system encouraging the elimination of toxins.
* Excellent for all skin types due to its ability to balance sebum. Useful for congested, dry, inflamed, oily or combination skin, burns, eczema, herpes and wounds.

Geranium is one of the most highly effective oils for the menopause and PMS – balancing the hormones, reducing fluid and alleviating tension.

Special precautions
None.

Jasmine

Latin name: *Jasminum officinale*
Family: OLEACEAE
Keywords: aphrodisiac, euphoric, healing, strengthening

Principal properties and effects

Jasmine is often referred to as the 'King of essential oils' and is frequently adulterated due to its high price.

* Invaluable for treating depression, inducing feelings of optimism, confidence and euphoria. Useful for apathy and indifference.
* Highly effective in childbirth, promoting the contractions yet inducing relaxation and relieving the pain. It promotes the flow of breast milk after the birth and prevents post-natal depression.
* Beneficial for all skin types especially dry, sensitive skin. Useful for stretch marks and scars and for increasing the elasticity of the skin.

Jasmine is a renowned aphrodisiac, jasmine alleviates premature ejaculation, frigidity and impotence. It strengthens the male sex organs and increases the sperm count.

Special precautions
Do not take internally.

Juniper

Latin name: *Juniperus communis*
Family: CUPRESSACEAE
Keywords: antiseptic, detoxifying, fluid reducing, purifying

Principal properties and effects

* A classic remedy for urinary infections such as cystitis. Excellent for relieving fluid retention and for those who have difficulty in passing urine.
* Effective for arthritis, gout and rheumatic disorders, stimulating the elimination of uric acid and other toxins.
* Indicated for acne, blocked pores, oily and congested skin, purifying and encouraging detoxification.

Juniper is renowned for its detoxifying and purifying ability. Juniper clears waste from the body as well as from the mind. Helpful for obesity, and after too much rich food and alcohol. An ideal oil for emotional depletion clearing and strengthening the mind.

Special precautions

* Avoid during pregnancy.
* Do not use excessively where there is inflammation of the kidneys.

Lavender

Latin name: *Lavandula officinalis/vera/angustifolia*
Family: LAMIACEAE (or Labiatae)
Keywords: analgesic, antidepressant, balancing, healing, rejuvenating, soothing

Principal properties and effects

* Highly recommended for the nervous system, relieving depression, anxiety and insomnia. Balances mood swings

and soothes anger, frustration and irritability. Useful for shock.
* Helpful for high blood pressure, palpitations and other cardiac disorders.
* Invaluable for pain relief in conditions such as arthritis, lumbago, rheumatism, sprains and strains.
* Renowned as an immune system booster; lavender is recommended for all infections and viruses, catarrh, colds and throat disorders.
* Excellent for all skin care due to its powers of rejuvenation and balancing effects. Helps to heal burns, sunburn, acne, boils, bruises, eczema, psoriasis and wounds and sores of all descriptions.

Lavender is one of the most popular and versatile essential oils used in aromatherapy. Its aroma is familiar to almost everyone and it is well established as a remedy for relaxation.

Special precautions

None. A gentle essential oil suitable for all ages from babies to the elderly.

Lemon

Latin name:	*Citrus limonum*
Family:	**RUTACEAE**
Keywords:	**alkaline, antiseptic, purifying, revitalizing, stimulant**

Principal properties and effects

* Highly recommended for the digestive system, particularly for counteracting acidity.
* Indicated for all infectious diseases; lemon boosts the immune system, reduces high temperatures and restores vitality, accelerating recovery time.

* Popular for skin care. Its cleansing action makes it suitable for oily skin (and hair), cuts and infected wounds, warts and verrucae.
* Stimulating for the circulatory system, liquefying the blood. Helpful for varicose veins (together with cypress) – gentle effleurage only.

To treat warts dab a drop of lemon onto the affected area with a cotton wool bud several times a day.

Special precautions

Avoid strong sunlight immediately after treatment.

Neroli (orange blossom)

Latin name:	*Citrus aurantium var. amara*
Family:	**RUTACEAE**
Keywords:	**antidepressant, aphrodisiac, rejuvenating, tranquillizing**

Principal properties and effects

* Effective for colic, colitis, diarrhoea and nervous indigestion.
* Recommended for reducing scarring and the prevention of stretch marks. Neroli is beneficial for all skin types, encouraging the regeneration of skin cells, particularly dry, mature and sensitive skin.
* Due to its aphrodisiac properties, effective for sexual problems such as impotence and frigidity.

Neroli is one of the most effective oils for the treatment of stress. It relieves chronic or short-term anxiety, soothes hysteria and shock and induces sleep.

Special precautions

None. A very gentle oil.

Peppermint

Latin name: *Mentha piperita*
Family: LAMIACEAE (or Labiatae)
Keywords: analgesic, cooling, digestive, pain relieving,
                 stimulating

Principal properties and effects

* Exerts a powerful effect on the digestive system.
  Recommended for sickness, diarrhoea and constipation.
  Relieves pain and spasm in the stomach and colon.
* Its pain-relieving properties make it invaluable for
  headaches and migraine, particularly if related to digestion.
  Highly effective for reducing muscular aches, neuralgia and
  rheumatism.
* Useful for stimulating the mind, eliminating mental fatigue
  and encouraging clarity of thought.
* Cools down sunburn and inflammation. Helpful for toxic
  congested skin, acne and oily skin.

Peppermint is often used to combat nausea – especially travel
sickness. Put a couple of drops on a tissue and inhale whenever
necessary.

Special precautions

* Store away from homoeopathic medications.
* Take care with sensitive skins – use in low concentrations.
* Avoid when breast feeding as it discourages the flow of
  breast milk.
* Do not use on babies and young children.

Rose

Latin name: *Rosa centifolia/damascena*
Family: ROSACEAE
Keywords: antidepressant, aphrodisiac, lingering and
                 loving, rejuvenating

Principal properties and effects

* The exquisite, luxurious aroma of rose has a profound effect on the emotions, filling the heart with love and alleviating depression, grief, jealousy, resentment, shock and tension.
* An invaluable oil for all female problems, regulating the menstrual cycle and cleansing and toning the womb. Helpful for PMS and the menopause. Recommended for frigidity, impotence and other sexual difficulties.
* Excellent for all types of skin, particularly dry, mature and sensitive skin. Reduces broken thread veins.

There are two types of rose oil available – rose otto and rose absolute. Rose otto, extracted by distillation, is of a superior quality.

Special precautions

None. Invaluable for women and gentle enough for use on children.

Rosemary

Latin name:	*Rosmarinus officinalis*
Family:	LAMIACEAE (or Labiatae)
Keywords:	analgesic, detoxifying, fluid reducing, restorative, stimulating

Principal properties and effects

* An invaluable restorative for loss of function, reviving muscles, limbs, memory, hair, smell and so forth.
* Highly recommended for pain relief in muscles and joints, easing arthritis, gout, rheumatism and stiff, overworked muscles.
* Beneficial for a wide range of digestive complaints where detoxification is required as with constipation, flatulence and liver congestion.
* Useful for combating fluid retention and lymphatic congestion. Effective for cellulite and obesity.
* Beneficial for the hair and scalp, encouraging hair growth and alleviating dandruff.

Rosemary activates and enlivens the brain, clearing the head and reducing mental fatigue. An ideal oil to use when studying.

Special precautions
Do not use excessively in pregnancy or in cases of epilepsy.

Sandalwood

Latin name: *Santalum album*
Family: SANTALACEAE
Keywords: aphrodisiac, healing, relaxing, uplifting

Principal properties and effects

* Well known for its balancing effects on the nervous system, gently soothing away anxiety and tension. Sandalwood engenders feelings of peace and tranquillity.
* Particularly valuable for urinary infections, alleviating cystitis and vaginal discharges of all kinds.
* Helpful for sexual problems such as impotence and frigidity.

Sandalwood is particularly beneficial for dry, cracked, chapped or dehydrated skin. When blended with a carrier oil it makes an excellent aftershave.

Special precautions
None.

Tea tree

Latin name: *Melaleuca alternifolia*
Family: MYRTACEAE
Keywords: antiseptic, anti-fungal, anti-infectious, stimulating

Principal properties and effects

* Renowned for its remarkable activity against bacteria, fungi and viruses and as a powerful immunostimulant, tea tree is a must for the first-aid kit in every household. Particularly